Homoeopathy
and Your Emotions

By the same author

Help Your Child with
Homeopathy

SHEILA HARRISON RGN

Homoeopathy
and Your Emotions

ASHGROVE PRESS, BATH

First published in Great Britain by
ASHGROVE PRESS LIMITED
4 Brassmill Centre, Brassmill Lane
Bath BA1 3JN

and distributed in the USA by
Avery Publishing Group Inc.
120 Old Broadway
Garden City Park
New York 11040

ISBN 1 85398 026 9

First published 1993

Typeset by Ann Buchan (Typesetters), Middlesex
Printed and bound in Great Britain by
Dotesios Ltd, Trowbridge, Wiltshire

Contents

HOMOEOPATHY

The rather strange and clumsy word 'homoeopathy' is
derived from the Greek words 'homoios' meaning 'like'
and 'pathos' meaning 'suffering'; so translated means
'like suffering', and homoeopathy then is the medical
practice of treating like with like. This is the basic or
fundamental law of homoeopathy which was expressed
by Samuel Hahnemann, the great German physician,
(1755–1843) as 'similia similibus curentur' – likes may be
cured by likes. This principle was well known to the
physicians of ancient times, Hippocrates and Paracelsus,
but was revised and built upon by Hahnemann in the
early part of the nineteenth century. He confirmed the
remarkable fact that a substance could cure the ailment
which it could cause. This principle has found its way
into modern usage in the phrase 'the hair of the dog that
bit you'. Numerous examples can be quoted to prove this
principle to be effective. If quinine is given to a healthy
person in fairly large quantities, most of the symptoms of
the disease malaria will arise, i.e. violent headache, buzz-
ing in the ears, aching of the limbs, etc. Now quinine is
the recognised remedy for malaria, and modern treat-
ments for malaria have been developed from this basic
plant material. In a similar way white arsenic produces
intense abdominal pain, diarrhoea and vomiting, and
Arsen. Alb. in homoeopathic potency is often the treatment of choice for this condition. Those who work with
radium and X-ray therapy in the treatment of cancer take
great care to avoid over-exposure to radiation themselves, as over-exposure can lead to the development of
cancerous growths. Another example of the principle of
like curing like is found in the use of Coffea which is often

7

given for sleeplessness by the homoeopath, whereas it is well-known that drinking too much coffee before bed-time will keep a person awake.

Hahnemann was so appalled by the medical practices of his day which often involved violent purging and blood-letting so severe that on occasions the patient died as a result of it, that he determined to seek a gentler form of approach. He, his students and his family set out to investigate the herbs and drugs which were later to form the basis of the homoeopathic Materia Medica of today – the list of remedies that are used to treat disease. These investigations were carried out by Hahnemann and his followers, by taking small quantities of known drugs and minerals for a period of time, often quite a long period of time, and noting the symptoms that arose as a result of taking those drugs. Patients who suffered from similar symptoms to those that had been produced in the experi-menter were then treated with tiny quantities of these substances and it was found that in many cases a com-plete cure of their illnesses resulted. These experiments were called 'provings' and are still carried out today on a somewhat limited scale by groups of homoeopaths all over the world who are still prepared to subject them-selves to uncomfortable experiences in order to find new and valuable remedies for the treatment of their patients.

Much has always been made of the fact that homoeopaths use tiny, even infinitesimal doses, of the remedy that they have chosen. Hahnemann's earlier experiments involved giving small but material doses of the remedies involved, but he discovered that often the therapeutic value of the remedies was enhanced if even smaller amounts were given; an additional benefit of the very small quantities of course was that the likelihood of side effects appearing was reduced.

Hahnemann then experimented with ways of carrying out this dilution and the method called 'succussion' or 'potentisation' was eventually developed and is still used to this day. This process consists of dilution of mineral or drug solution again and again with violent shaking, the diluent usually used being a solution of pure alcohol. Whilst it was found that the highly diluted solution of the correct remedy was very effective in use, if the wrong remedy was chosen in error it had no effect whatsoever, so the patient was safe and protected from side effects. It is this astonishing effect of the minute dose that has lead to the strongest criticisms of homoeopathy, criticisms that the homoeopaths have found most difficult to answer. The cry has so often been, 'there is no scientific proof', and the accusation is often made that cures are due to the placebo effect, that the patient gets better because he believes he will. In all systems of medicine this is a factor that cannot be ignored, and the bedside manner has always been important in the establishment of trust between physician and patient. However, this criticism of homoeopathy falls down when one considers its use with animals and infants where the patient does not even know that what is being administered is a medicine. In recent times double blind trials, so beloved of the drug companies, have been carried out on homoeopathic remedies and these trials have proved those remedies to be effective beyond question. The proof of the pudding however is in the eating and homoeopaths are usually too busy helping people to get well to be interested in denying them treatment for the benefit of scientific research, so for this reason much of homoeopathic reporting is anecdotal.

The homoeopath is concerned with assessing the person as a whole rather than the disease as a set of symptoms, which he sees as the body's reaction to the illness, and will be extremely interested in the person's mental as well as physical make-up, whether their colouring is dark or fair, whether they are better for movement or quiet, better in the morning or the evening, better in cold or hot weather; all these things are pointers to the correct remedy, in addition to a knowledge of the patient's past medical history, particularly of past infectious illness. When the remedy is chosen and administered its effect is to stimulate the body's own in-built healing ability to overcome the disease in order that symptoms are no longer created and physical and mental harmony are restored.

Fortunately for our purpose there is a large group of homoeopathic remedies referred to as the 'Polycrests' which are given in the same tiny doses as before, but which can be chosen very simply without the long and complicated case-taking that the professional homoeopath applies. It is these remedies that form the basis of many self-help books on homoeopathy.

HOW TO SELECT THE REMEDY

As you will see from the account of the remedies, symptoms of anxiety, depression, hysteria, moroseness, suicidal tendencies, and mania may be found, within the same remedy. Homoeopathy does not give labels to mental illness because it is potentially impractical to do so.

Each remedy can be roughly divided into three stages. The first stage of a remedy can be seen with the symptoms in their mildest form, with the bulk of the later symptoms absent.

The individual may never become a patient at all, but go through life being a nuisance to themselves, and other people, but never becoming really ill. It is only when the stresses of life begin to weigh on them that they may move into the second stage and start to show signs of instability.

Let us consider Aurum Metallicum as the example remedy as we work through the process.

We see the basic Aurum personality, responsible, and hard working, with a strong desire to 'do the right thing'. This type of person will irritate his less concientious work mates no doubt, as he will be a stickler for detail, and not go home until he has balanced the books and left everything in good order for the next day. He will make sure that the in-trays have been cleared, that messages have not been overlooked and that the office door has been locked. Then and only then will he be satisfied that he can go home to his orderly life and an evening of classical music to relax him.

He has met a nice girl, usually his opposite, outgoing, casual, and good company, and contemplating matrimony will decide to go into business for himself. After all he has all the attributes to succeed, since he is by nature an achiever.

His business starts well, for he leaves no stone unturned, and with the wedding over everything is set fair for the future. However, his wife becomes pregnant and the government juggles the economy imposing some unforeseen problems on his business, and we are set to move into the second phase – we have a potential patient. However, you won't get your hands on him at this stage, more's the pity, because if you could a great deal of trouble could be saved.

Now his business is in difficulty and he has responsibilities, so the next stage is anxiety. Anxious that things are going wrong, that he will not be able to do as well for his dependants as he had hoped, he arrives home irritable.

His wife senses the tension in him and prepares his favourite meal. He can't control his anxiety, neither can he bring himself to sit down and talk about the difficulties, since he is afraid of failing, so he will find something to pick and complain about.

He will be irritable and ready to find fault with his wife's housekeeping, or her appearance, anything to discharge his anxiety. If this goes on for any length of time, depending who he has married, he will find himself with a bewildered and resentful wife, who is doing her best to please and is beginning to feel as though she is having to bring up the family without any support from her husband.

If she can get him to the marriage guidance service, she will be very lucky. After all, he is doing all the right things. He is working all the hours that God sends, providing her with a good home. What more can she want? She, by this time, is beginning to think that the whole business of being married is a disaster and not worth the candle.

Secretly, he is beginning to feel that he has let his loved ones down and is no use to them at all, life is not worth living, and depression sets in. It is just possible now that he will go to the Doctor for help, and this, if you are lucky, is when you will get him, at the end of the second stage.

It only needs now for his wife to leave him, or a lull in his business, and he will be tipped over the edge. He has done his best, yet everything has gone wrong. He feels defeated and unworthy and may suddenly commit suicide without warning. He does not threaten to do away with himself – he will just do it.

This progression applies to all remedies, and it is unlikely that patients will present for treatment until they are at the end of the second stage, or even well into the third stage, so in selecting the remedy what has gone before is all important. So often in the third stage of mental illness one remedy picture can be very much like another, so it is important to go back and build up over a period of time to help select the correct remedy.

Another common scenario is the good student who has worked hard and consistently all the way through University. The last year, in an effort to get high honours, he will become anxious and push himself too far. Having burned himself out just before his finals he may get lower grades than he had expected, and without warning kill himself, leaving family and friends completely bewildered as to his motive.

You will see as you read through the remedies how easy it is to divide each picture into the three stages.

Having found the correct remedy, administer it in the 200c potency and await events. When improvement has stopped, repeat the chosen remedy in a high potency such as 1M, and again wait. When improvement stops, check to see that the chosen remedy is still the right one, as the case may have changed and another remedy may be indicated. If this is not the case proceed into higher potencies 10M, 50M or 10MM. Give one dose and wait.

When improvement has stopped it will be necessary to re-take the case if the results are not completely satisfactory, and a new prescription may be necessary. The reason for this is that people do not go through life with the same personality traits, they change. When the acute condition has been cured you will have taken them back to the stage they were in previously. If any abberations that are left can be treated, then success is assured.

IF THE INDICATED REMEDY FAILS TO WORK

There are a number of reasons why the chosen remedy may not work, or have only limited success. More often than not the reason is that the wrong one has been chosen, either because the therapist has missed a vital clue, or the patient has been misleading. It is all too easy to dismiss a chance remark which will lead to the right indication.

It is a good idea to have a homoeopathic prescriber to hand when selecting the remedy, to look up any physical symptoms the patient might have; then, when comparing the remedies, pointers can be gained in helping the choice.

Vaccination and immunisation can cause blockages in the body, preventing the indicated remedy from working. Where will we find anybody these days who has not had one or another inflicted upon them? In these cases a dose of Thuja 200, followed a few weeks later by the indicated remedy, can work wonders.

Thuja helps to antidote the miasms that have been inflicted on the patient by the injection of foreign proteins at the time of vaccination or immunisation. Very often the symptom picture will change after the Thuja and may have to be taken again.

Suppression of pus must also be taken into consideration. Often a young person will become schizophrenic after prolonged treatment with antibiotics for pustular acne,and until suitable remedies for pustular eruptions have been administered, and the old condition brought out again, there will be no cure.

Also supression of any skin ailments by cortisone therapy will have a similar effect. The affinity between the brain and the skin often goes unnoticed, in spite of the fact that their development in utero are synonymous.

The best way to deal with this situation is to make every effort to deal with the physical condition prior to the onset of mental disturbance. In many cases the mental symptoms will disappear or at least be modified, and of course a new prescription will be necessary.

Miasms can also block the expected improvement and must be considered. Generally speaking most people these days have a fairly equal distribution of the four miasms, although some have one predominant. If the predominaant miasm is very obvious, a dose of the 200c potency of its nosode will help to unlock the blockage.

Do not give Carcinosin, Luesticium, Medorrhinum or Tuberculin to a patient who has had a serious skin complaint if you are not a Homoeopath, as the complaint may re-occur and you will not be able to deal with it. Enlist the help of a homoeopath or herbalist to deal with the skin complaint first.

Allergic symptoms can distort the mental picture too, as certain foods have been identified as being particularly prone to aggravate the brain. Grains, more particularly wheat, dairy products, coffee, sugar and food colourings are among the most common of these. If any of these foods can be considered suspect, a week of abstaining from them may be very revealing. Skin scratch allergy testing is notoriously inaccurate on foodstuffs, but more accurate on airborne materialsl such as house dust and animal hairs. Thyroid dysfunction mainly in women must also be taken into consideration and treated where necessary as the problem may ease or disappear after treatment.

Mercury sensitivity may also be a problem, as some people are very sensitive to the amalgam fillings in their teeth. Amalgam and gold fillings in the same mouth cause electrical discharges to take place which I have found interfere with the energy of the remedy and cause a poor response.

Mercury is leached out over the years and swallowed by the patient, the mercury then becoming fixed in the tissues, causing mercurial poisoning. A first aid antidote may be administered; either Merc.Sol, or Hepar Sulph. on a daily basis while the problem is investigated and dealt with.

Hypoglycaemia must also be considered and treated, as the mood swings in this condition can be almost as bad in severe cases as manic depressive psychosis. Certain shortages can also be a problem in some patients especially the B. Vitamins or Zinc, so clear questioning about the diet is always important as many people these days though consuming vast quantities of food may be suffering from simple malnutrition and overdosing of food additives. The body chemistry is very important, vitamins, minerals, and amino acids being the corner stones of the body chemistry. The brain must have the correct food if it is to function properly, as the chemistry of the brain governs our whole existence.

There are plenty of good books to be had on these subjects, some of which will be recommended at the end of this book.

THE THYROID GLAND

The consequences of thyroid dysfunction are very often overlooked by psychiatrists, psychologists and general practitioners.

There is a good reason for this, as during a ten minute consultation consisting of a list of emotional difficulties, the first thought is to prescribe psychiatric drugs to see if they help, and the second course is to refer to a psychiatrist.

Thyroid dysfunction, however, plays a very important part in the mental processes, particularly in women at puberty, childbirth and the menopause.

Psychiatrists and psychotherapists have left the soma behind and become immersed in Freud, Jung, Adler and company, often completely overlooking the endocrine system. An unbalanced thyroid gland will produce an unbalanced patient. The sales of Valium would plummet if more attention were paid to balancing thyroid function.

Thyroid tests may come back from the laboratory within normal limits, but what is considered to be within the criteria laid down may not be acceptable for a particular patient in order to function well. Much can be done to balance the Thyroid homoeopathically and with supplements.

The main function of the gland is to produce thyroxin, the consumption of which is 1/2–1 milligram daily. Thyroxin contains 67% iodine: therefore shortage of iodine impairs production.

HYPERTHYROIDISM (Thyrotoxicosis)

Excessive production of normal secretion
The size of the gland may increase
Protruding eyes Loss of weight
Fine tremor in hands
Palpitation and tachycardia
General nervous irritability
More common in women than men. (6 – 1)
Panic Attacks
Family susceptibility
Onset is most common between puberty and 35 years
May be brought on by nervous shock; childbirth
Invariably symptoms of rheumatism
Gallstones or liver disruptions
Anaemia

The onset may be sudden which is usually the case in primary thyrotoxicosis, but may be insidious in adenoma.

The adenomatus state may be present for years without being recognised and hospital tests will show thyroid activity within normal limits. Thus the patient will suffer without treatment and may be dubbed a neurotic or fall out with her family, who think she is just being awkward.

This condition may persist and, unless the gland becomes actively toxic, may never be properly diagnosed.

The gland is usually enlarged, but if it is not diagnosis is made more difficult.

The degree of increase in size of the gland has no relationship to the severity of the symptoms, in fact the gland may be very large with only mild symptoms, and vice versa.

The Heart and circulation alter during the progress of the disease. Palpitation and tachycardia are among the first symptoms. The apex beat may be so forcible as to shake the patient. There may be pulsation even in capillaries.

If allowed to continue, unrecognised enlargement of the heart will follow.

Nervous System	Patients become altered mentally
	Cross
	Irritable
	Unpredictable
	Suicidal
	Homicidal
	Exhilarated one day, exhausted the next – even from hour to hour
Eyes	Exophthalmus occurs in 70% of cases
Stellway's Sign	Infrequent and incomplete blinking
Von Groefe's Sign	Eyelids lag behind movements of eyes
Joffrey's Sign	On looking towards ceiling with face inclined downwards, forehead does not wrinkle
Bullet's Sign	Loss of eye movement without loss of pupil reaction
Moebius' Sign	On attempting to focus on a close object one eye turns outwards

Metabolism   Increased rate in combustion of
                        food. If appetite and absorption
                        not good – rapid loss of weight,
                        although every case does not lose
                        weight. Proteins are broken up
                        very rapidly. Oxidation of
                        carbohydrates is modified and
                        may produce glycosurea.

HYPOTHYROIDISM MYXOEDEMA
(underproduction of the hormone)

Often found in members of the same family
Loss of memory
Lack of concentration
Pains near joints without rheumatic or neurotic
character
Skin tends to be dry and harsh
Baggy eyelids
Hair goes thin and outer edge of eyebrows may drop
out
Legs may appear oedematus but no pitting on
pressure
Hands become clumsy and spadelike
Feels the cold even when quite warm atmosphere
Difficulty making decisions
Metabolism low with temperature below normal
Poor appetite and constipation with weight gain
Weakness in legs
Clumsy walking

Disruption of the thyroid can often be attributed to
pregnancy, as the thyroid tends to enlarge from the 5th
month although no symptoms of thyroid dysfunction are

obvious. This normally settles down after the birth, but many cases can be traced to pregnancy.

So if a patient presents with any of the symptoms of thyroid dysfunction after pregnancy, it would be well to watch them carefully and if necessary treat. A week of homoeopathic iodine may be all that is required, or, alternatively, 1 dose of 3 drops Thyroid 200 could be enough to normalise the gland.

A condition of sub-thyroid malfunction may manifest itself.

In these cases, the patient may have alternating symptoms of over or under activity changing from day to day or even alongside one another.

This condition is very difficult to recognise and care should be taken to watch carefully before prescribing.

I have developed a rule of thumb treatment which is effective.

Blue eyed, fair skinned – Spongia 12c twice daily until stable to be repeated as necessary.

Dark hair with light eyes – Calcium Iodide in the same dosage.

Dark hair, dark skin and eyes – Iodine in the same dosage.

In more severe cases, Thyroid 1x – 3 times daily until stabilised. This dosage will get good results in either hyperthyroidism or hypothyroidism.

There is usually an imbalance of Potassium, Magnesium, and Calcium in these patients and a supplement of these minerals along with Vitamin B will usually help to keep them balanced. The lifestyle of these patients should be examined as prolonged stress, such as an unhappy marriage or a frustrated life, if not cleared up, will cause constant regression in the treatment.

Sexual problems are common, which of course could lead to distressing mental troubles. Infertility, gynaecological complaints and miscarriages, and lack of sexual desire are all pointers to thyroid imbalance which, if not rectified, lead to untold mental distress and the breakdown of relationships.

THE MIASMS OF HAHNEMANN

In order fully to understand the fundamentals of inherited tendencies you need to have a basic grasp of the theory of the miasms.

Samuel Hahnemann believed that there were three main constitutional diseases, which he called miasms, but present day meanings have altered as a better understanding of genetical influences have come under the microscope.

A miasm is a constitutional state, caused by either the suppression of disease by drug therapy, or an inherited stigma from the acute diseases of previous generations. When these stigmata are present very often the Homoeopathic remedy, even when strongly indicated, will fail to act. So it is very important to be able to recognise the stigma (miasm) in your patient.Most people today have all the stigmata, but in some patients one or more of the stigmata are outstanding and must be treated if complete success is to be accomplished.

Hahnemann stated that the original stigma came from leprosy and called it Psora. The next great diseases of man which followed were Syphillis and Gonorrhoea. Psora and Syphilis combined, causing a predisposition to the next great scourge in the form of Tuberculosis, and this has since been followed by Cancer, combining all the miasms – Psora, Syphilis, Gonorrhoea and Tuberculosis.

This does not mean that everybody with all the stigmata will necessarily develop cancer, but should the Vital

Life Force of the body become deranged the possibility is greater.

Emotional shock is the most common cause of this happening, although the stress of severe virus infections and accidents can have the same effect.

The miasms or stigmata are the basis of all chronic disease as they disorganise the whole system, both physically and mentally.

It is clear then that should a particular miasm be predominant, it may be necessary to give priority to that miasm and give a few doses of its nosode to be followed by the indicated remedy.

PSORA (the leprosy miasm)

The psoric patient has a quick brain and is constantly involved in mental activity, which tires him out. Psorics are anxious and filled with foreboding. They always expect the worst and are afraid that they are ill when they are not, or that any illness they may have is much more serious than it is, or may even be fatal. They have periods of sadness and dread physical work, but will have bursts of energy followed by prostration. Anxiety often appears at the full moon, especially during menstruation; they feel better after a good cry. The psoric miasm often has palpitations and tremblings, may be extremely nervous, perspiration is often profuse and ameliorates symptoms. Fear is a great symptom; they fear the dark, an ordeal, crowds, the future, anything. They are never calm and peaceful, but always too much aware of their surroundings and hypersensitive to everything. They have great powers of understanding and are quick on the uptake, but unable to use all their knowledge to good effect since they cannot sustain their efforts. If they make themselves sustain them, eventually they will collapse. They can be fast talking and full of theories, always theorising, ana-lysing themselves and other people. Never satisfied with anything for long, they are always searching for some-thing that will satisfy them, but never quite know what. They are very often prone to liver troubles. The emotional disturbances from which the psoric patient suffers cause malfunctions and non-structural changes. Psora on its own never causes structural changes, and must be com-bined with another miasm in order to do so. The psoric patient has problems of assimilation and does not get out of his food all the nutrients he needs. This encourages deficiency diseases which in turn aggravate the situation. They are always hungry, even after food, have cravings for unusual savoury or sweet food, and like highly spiced food. The psoric feels full quickly but is soon hungry again.

LUETISUM (the syphillis miasm)

Although a disease of 500 years standing, allopathic methods have only ever served partially to cure syphilis. Unfortunately, the symptoms do not appear until the disease has already caused havoc. Consequently, the miasm is passed from generation to generation since it causes cellular abormality. In all its forms it is a very deep-seated disease and the miasm thus causes deep-seated changes in the body. Mental symptoms of the syphilitic miasm are dullness, stupidity, slowness, fixed ideas, suspicion, fixed moods, difficulty in understand-ing, frustration, and slow powers of reasoning. There are usually eye and ear problems, poor bone structure in the nose, mis-shapen palate and teeth. The syphilitic miasm likes cold food and drink, and has an aversion to meat.

SYCOSIS (the gonorrhoeal miasm)

This only manifests itself in future generations if it has not been completely cured and has been suppressed. If this is the case, the aftermath will be inflammation of joints, muscles, and malfunction of the lymphatic system. It tends to attack the female reproductive organs with overgrowth of tissue, e.g. fibroids, polyps. In the male it leads to kidney and prostate troubles. Sycotic miasm is cross and irritable especially when there are changes in the weather, is very suspicious even of himself, always assumes that he has been misunderstood, assumes that everyone else is suspicious and as mistrustful as he is, is very jealous, secretive, tends to check his work, often tells lies in order to vindicate himself, is likely to be cruel to animals, deceitful, unable to give affection or appreciate it from others, and likely to have fits of anger. He tends to crave beer, fat meat and sauces. Infants with this miasm usually suffer from colic from birth to three months, and often there is a great deal of wind which is expelled violently.

PSEUDO-PSORA (the combined miasm of psora and syphilis) TUBERCULOSIS

The person tends to be unsociable, sullen, morose, the children having learning difficulties and being slow in comprehension. There is a tendency to hysteria. The appearance of the eyes is characteristic: they often have a bluish translucent appearance around and beneath the them. They usually have a craving for salt, long for stimulants and exotic food, crave meat and potatoes, enjoy extremely hot or very cold foods, often feel faint with hunger and usually have no appetite for breakfast. They may have a desire for a particular food and then when it is available they do not want it. The tubercular miasm is always present in hernias. Breathing is shallow and there are often chest problems.

CARCINOSIN

The appearance of this patient can physically cover every shape and size; they may be excessively thin, or on the other hand obese, indicating metabolic disturbances.

There may be warts, moles and birthmarks and in fair complexions prominent veins, especially on the face and hands, or a dusky hue, described as the 'cafe au lait' complexion.

Fear is a prominent symptom, particularly fears with no exciting cause, and anxiety is very marked. They are very good at supressing their fears, but eventually when stressed by circumstances, they will bring their fears out in the open. They fear almost anything, and may be introverted, antisocial, anxious about trifles, afraid of illness – especially cancer – or afraid of insanity.

Irritability is also strong in these patients, they can be angry, rough, rude, destructive, cruel and uncontrollable. They themselves, although aware of their behaviour cannot control it, and will even manipulate situations so that they can have an outburst.

Because all the miasms are present in the cancer miasm the symptoms both mental and physical can be contradictory. They may be over fastidious or scruffy, very intelligent or dull, and so on.

Within the cancer miasm itself, you will be able to see a fair distribution of the other miasms, though one may appear pre-dominant.

The remedy (Carcinosin) will be useful when the case has been taken if no one remedy is marked, and there appears to be an overlap, as though one remedy picture is imposed on another. A dose of carcinosin 30c, 200c and 1M, administered in that order on the same day will be helpful. A waiting period of about 6 – 8 weeks if possible will bring changes in the patient, and it will then be much more clear when taking the case which remedy is the more suitable.

Insomnia is a common feature, particularly when there is no obvious cause. There may be periods of disturbed sleep.

Desires and aversions to certain foods, commonly fat, meat, milk, eggs, sweets and wines are helpful indications for this remedy.

Family history is important, as any of the following illnesses in the family indicate that this remedy would be beneficial: Cancer, Pernicious Anaemia, Leukaemia, Hyperplastic Anaemia, Aplastic Anaemia, Hodgkins Disease, Muscular Dystrophy, Rheumatoid Arthritis, Diabetes, Lupus erythematosis, Cirrhosis of the Liver, Emotional instability and mental disturbances, congenital abnormalities, and any of the degenerative diseases.

It is not considered advisable to give this nosode to any patient who has had cancer or has cancer. This advice also applies to any patient with Tuberculosis – do not give Tuberculin. In patients who have a well established degenerative disease, carcinosin should only be administered in the lower potencies, but in patients whose symptoms are of the mind, a single dose of a high potency may be given, even as high as 10M or 50M. It should not be repeated until the improvement has come to a standstill.

So, we can see a progression through the ages of the effects of deep-seated diseases that have spread throughout the world, building one on top of another to form a new disease and a new miasm. At the moment we are looking at a new disease in the form of A.I.D.S. which has so many characteristics of all the miasms, particularly Tuberculosis, but as yet there has been no Homoeopathic proving of the Aids virus, and therefore no nosode available.

ACUTE MANIA

The three main well-known remedies for acute mania are Belladonna, Hyoscyamus and Stramonium. The symptoms for these remedies do not progress noticeably through the three stages which I mentioned earlier but appear to be of sudden onset, and are unlikely to be seen outside a mental institution or psychiatric unit. However, there is always the first attack and should this occur before the patient is committed and the appropriate medicine given it will surely shorten their stay in hospital and may even avert the necessity for restraint and heavy drugging.

The patient who flips into an acute manic state has always been treatable with a constitutional remedy. An example of this is Belladonna. Belladonna is related to Calc.Carb and Sulphur and is the chronic of Calc.Carb. e.g. Calc.Carb. has hot head and cold feet, while Sulphur also has an unstable circulation with flushes of heat in the body, particularly the plump Sulphur patients. It is as well therefore to take the case from relatives if need be, in order to find the remedy that is required prior to the attack of acute mania and be prepared once the crisis is past to treat with that remedy.

Other remedies I have mentioned, if not treated, can reach a stage of mania but the onset of these manias is progressive so it is necessary in these cases too to consult relatives to help differentiate between the acute mania and the progressive mania which belongs to another remedy.

Mercurius is an example of this as the mania of Mercury resembles the others in many ways and can easily be mistaken in haste. Mercury poisoning is very common, often goes undetected and is well worth investigation. Amalgam fillings in the teeth can produce a proving of Mercury and certainly dentists and patients are becoming increasingly aware of this problem.

Hyoscyamus

Here, as in Belladonna, the patient is quite lively and vigorous by nature; again, headaches are a problem. The headaches are violent, heavy and long lasting. The head feels heavy and they are unable to think clearly. Headaches with pricking sensations, especially on the left side and on the crown: occipitial headaches and drawing pain in the nape of the neck, also a sensation of water in the head when waking.

They are very talkative and will turn out no end of rubbish to all and sundry with embarrassing personal information. Usually worse in the evening, they will pick quarrels and make out they are badly done to.

These patients are extremely anxious, restless and afraid. They will imagine somebody is there who is not, that they are going to be eaten by animals. Ridiculous behaviour is common, as are dancing, singing love songs, face pulling. They will scramble about in the bed in the most peculiar positions and will beat the bed rhythmically with the arm and pick at the bedclothes.

Their behaviour alternates between being placid, sad, and deep in thought to absolute fury. The fury is so great that restraint is necessary as they have a vice like grip and superhuman strength, and are quite capable of injuring somebody or themselves.

A strange feature of the remedy is that the patient will go through the motion of doing a job or preparing to go somewhere. Often they will complain that somebody has tried to poison them and they will not drink as they are afraid of water.

Vertigo, fainting, rigidity, hysteria, catatonic states and convulsions are common to the remedy.

Usually worse after eating, there is a lot of flatulence, and frequent bowel movement or even diarrhoea and prolonged bouts of hiccoughs and disturbances of vision.

The face is hot, especially the ear lobes, and brownish-red rather than the bright red of Belladonna, although the complexion can be bluish or earthy, as the circulation changes.

The sleep is restless and disturbed, and they will wake up with a start and cry out.

Stramonium

The Stramonium patient looks worried, worn and sad. Sad they are, very, very sad since they dwell on death and do a good deal of crying. They feel as though they have done something bad all the time. Afraid of the dark, they must have company and feel as though they have been abandoned if they don't get it. There is a fear of water, and the sound of running water makes them agitated. Lights reflecting in mirrors bother them too, because probably they look like water and bright lights bother them anyway.

They are voluble and inclined to babble on about all sorts of rubbish which drives people away, so then they are abandoned. If they get too excitable the face and ears become hot but the nose tends to stay pale.

Sleep is disturbed, with bad dreams, and they will grind their teeth and bang their head into the pillow. Stammering, jerky movements, stumbling, particularly in the dark, and a tendancy to face backwards and to the left are common symptoms. Under great stress they may even be unable to speak at all.

Not any easy remedy to spot in the early stages, but as they move into the next stage it may become more obvious. The fear of water is more marked and they will even back away from a cup of liquid and refuse to drink.

There is muttering and staring with a fixed stare as though seeing something of which they are afraid.

The face becomes red and the whole head looks heated and pupils dilate, in fact they look for all the world as though they are drunk.

The possibilities are legion, singing, shouting, fits of sardonic laughter, swearing, praying, either singly or together.

Preaching and raving like an evangelist expecting people to come and be saved. God speaks to them and they will prophesy. They will see ghosts and evil spirits.

Great fears are prominent. They will see black objects, people and animals, or a myriad of different insects swarming, dogs attacking them, trying to eat them.

They suffer fits from fright, one side paralysed, the other with chorea, the chorea having a graceful, flailing movement; foaming at the mouth and spitting, and incontinence of the bowel.

The patient may feel to be all shapes and sizes. They will strike, tear or even stab if they have a handy tool, they want to kill others and themselves. They will throw themselves about the floor, crawl like a dog and try to eat the floor or will pretend to be other animals and behave accordingly.

All these phenomena can be interspersed with an exaggerated attitude of being haughty and important, almost as though they are overacting a part and it could be almost amusing if the situation were not so fraught.

Belladonna

These patients have a good physique and ruddy complexion. They are intelligent and have plenty of go in them. They have an unstable circulation with hot head and cold feet and a tendency to high blood pressure.

Headaches are a problem for them. The headaches are worse for movement and open air but relieved by rest and quiet. The least jar will set them off. The headaches are throbbing, pulsating, or jerking, and they will often complain that the front of the brain feels cold or that there is liquid moving about in the head. It is odd that they should have this cold feeling in the head as the outstanding thing about Belladonna is the heat in the head. The face looks red and the whole head looks hot. Even the eyes are very bright and shiny.

They are sensitive to draughts, particularly to the head, and are headsore – they cannot bear having the hair combed.

The memory is impaired, they become forgetful and will spend ages looking for things, muttering all the while. Quite sensible during the day, they become worse at night when they will pick arguments.

There is great fear of imaginary things and they will see ghosts, monsters, faces, insects and black dogs, and will appear terrified if you go near them

So terrified are they that they will attack themselves and others, given the chance. The rage and fury are uncontrollable except by restraint. They will rip, tear, spit, throw things, real or imaginary, and will gnaw through objects like a dog and may even bark like one.

On the other hand, they may strip off their clothes and start singing and dancing, pulling hideous faces and putting out the tongue for all the world like somebody who is drunk.

In between these manic phases they may lapse into a stage of being morose, weepy, fearful and extremely serious and become so apathetic that nothing will interest them at all.

31

MATERIA MEDICA

Anacardium

This remedy is often useful in schizophenia, though it is not confined to this condition.

These patients have a poor memory and even loss of memory. They have difficulty remembering what they need to know, but it comes to them later. Things seem unreal to them, and they can give the impression of being imbeciles. When talking to them they seem to understand what is being discussed, but later it becomes apparent that they have understood nothing, probably because they have forgotten the details of the discussion, although the impression one gets is that they are being obtuse.

There is a feeling of being two different people, one good and one bad. Degrees of this feeling can range from feeling good and bad to actually hearing angels telling him to do good and the devil telling him to do bad things. Swearing is common – and he hears the devil encouraging him to swear, do bad things and even commit murder. Angels can also command him to do bad things in the guise of doing good. An example of this type of situation can be seen in people who murder prostitutes, because an angel told him to.

There seem to be two wills, one commanding and the other forbidding.

This patient is very suspicious and is afraid of everything and everybody, believing that they are his enemies. Usually because he has very fixed ideas he will have one or two enemies who he believes are constantly out to do him down, so we see the paranoid personality here.

They are lacking in confidence and believe that they can accomplish nothing. Sulky and sullen they take everything the wrong way, and can become violent.

Very often they believe that their relatives or family are not theirs or that their children don't belong to them. This can be a temporary condition after childbirth when the mother denies she has had a baby.

Fortunately, in these particular cases the condition doesn't last long. In a Sepia patient there will be disinterest in the child, but in Anacardium there will be outright denial.

Often they have the feeling that they don't belong to this world and because everything seems unreal to them they will laugh at serious situations. The vision can be unclear and objects appear to be a long way off.

Very often these patients are convinced that there is somebody with them or that they are two people. These phases alternate with rational periods when, although they have illusions they are conscious these are not true.

Argent. Nit.

Although this is a remedy commonly associated with anxiety these patients may, in the later stages, show signs of being depressive and feel deep despair.

The appear to be hyperactive most of the time, which eventually exhausts them and everybody associated with them. This period of exhaustion can be misleading, as they appear to be depressed to the point of melancholia.

A constant state of apprehension is the norm for these people. They feel that they will never get anything done that must be done, yet time passes slowly.

Fear of meeting new people is common, as is a constant fear of failure. The 'what if' syndrome is also very prominent. 'What if we are late' or 'what if there is an accident?'. They imagine the worst always and if reassured then the 'yes but' syndrome surfaces. 'Yes but the plane may crash' or 'yes but the boat may sink', etc. and ad nauseam. There is no reassurance possible as they will always find a new possibility to worry about.

This abnormal level of anxiety can cause physical symptoms, such as sweating, sudden outbursts of temper, fluctuating blood pressure, and loss of muscle tone so that the body trembles and may even collapse, as the knees give way.

Chest pains are common as are tinnitus, pains in the head, diarrhoea, and claustrophobia, particularly in crowded places.

There is fear of heights, both looking up as well as looking down, and they may feel as though high buildings are coming down on them. There is the fear of wanting to jump from high buildings or into water from a bridge, and they may actually do it, although usually their legs give way and they will crumple to the ground.

In the later stages they can become quite irrational, with sudden ideas which they must put into operation at once. These can be obsessions, phobias, impulsive behaviour, hallucinations, loss of memory, fear of death, and a sudden impulse to commit suicide. Sometimes they will even predict when they are going to die.

Arsen. Alb.

The Arsen Alb patient is generally physically of fine
structure: neat, clean and of good bearing. They wear
well chosen clothes with a good colour sense. Women
will have hat, shoes and handbag to match and tone with
their outfit. They are very choosy when out shopping and
will not settle for something that will just do. It must be
right. They will want to know exactly what medication
they are having and why, then check over everything you
have said, almost as though they want to catch you out,
but really they must be absolutely sure of what they are
getting. They will never exceed the stated dose, and even
harmless medicines are carefully put out of harm's way.
They would never eat anything after the sell-by date.

They are, however, very restless people, always a bit
anxious and these anxieties can get out of hand and
become very stressful to them. There is a desire to have
somebody to talk to all the time, and if they have, then
they can forget their fears temporarily. There is fear of
the dark and their mental symptoms are always worse at
night. They will be out of bed wandering about the house
at night; after all if, they are awake nothing can happen
while they are asleep. They are great door lockers because they fear being broken into.

When ill, they don't really expect to get better and will
say that there seems little point in taking the medicine as
it can't really do much for them. However, once per-
suaded, they will take it religiously.

There is a feeling that they have done something bad
for which there can be no forgiveness or that they have

caused offence to others and in extreme circumstances they believe their sins to be so bad that there is no hope and become tormented with religious thoughts.

They believe the police are coming for them, that there are rats and mice in the bedroom and they will try to hide. Maniacal states may ensue, with screaming, crying, moaning and grinding of teeth, after which they relapse into a quiet state.

There is always a danger of suicide when the quiet phase comes or just when you think the worst is over.

Aurum

The patient who will eventually need Aurum starts out in life as a conscientious type of person. They are the kind of person who is intelligent, careful, prudent, a stickler for doing things right and very responsible in their attitudes to life. Usually they are set on the road to illness by grief, disappointment in love, shock or failure to achieve what they feel it is their duty to achieve.

A businessman whose business fails or an employee being made redundant or sacked for some minor mistake is liable to fall prey to the failure syndrome.

They lose hope and they lose their instinct for self-preservation. After all, they have done everything right; but their lives have gone wrong, therefore there seems no point. They lose their love of life and become weary of it.

Expectations are lowered and they feel that they will not succeed, and believe they have neglected their duties to family and friends and anything that goes wrong in their life is nothing more than they deserve because of their neglect. There is a feeling that they actually deserve to be punished, that they are unworthy and have done wrong. Depression can be so deep that they will sit and say nothing, and thoughts of death give them pleasure.

Generally, this patient will keep the way he feels to himself, and will commit suicide on impulse, taking everyone who knows him completely by surprise, as he was apparently of sound mind.

There is an angry side to this patient, too, which usually comes before the deep depression. They feel hateful, and can be worried over nothing, angry, with a flushed face and even violent. Obstinacy is marked, particularly if offers of help come their way, which can trigger angry outbursts.

An example of this kind of situation can be seen in the man who is struggling to get his business off the ground. He comes home looking tired and irritable. His family, sensing that all is not well, will try to please him, but for their pains will probably be bombasted or picked on and nothing will please him. The middle class businessman whose wife leaves him for mental cruelty or physical violence is ten to one an Aurum patient.

Mental exhaustion, eye problems, and digestive problems are common. They are very sensitive to noise, but music soothes them, particularly classical music and opera.

Calcium Carbonate

The Calc. Carb. type is generally plump, chilly and underactive. Their metabolism is slow due, no doubt, to the fact that their endocrine system tends to be underactive, especially the pituitary and thyroid glands. Their co-ordination is generally poor and they are generally a bit 'floppy', especially the handshake. If you hold their hand it feels like one that you have picked up somewhere. One feels that they are lazy but every effort tires them out. What is a normal day's work for many people is a big day's work for them.

'Off with the fairies' is my description of them, as they appear dreamy and seem to be taking no notice. They are slow learners, too, as everything is such an effort. They are forgetful about what they have just read, or conversations that have just taken place, probably because they haven't really been concentrating, yet they can surprise you by coming out with a remark which shows that they have really taken it all in. Also they never seem to have quite grown up – there is a child-like quality in their relationships. They are great gigglers and awful time-keepers.

They are sensitive – and will cry if chastised and they are also sensitive to others' misfortunes, as they imagine how they must be feeling.

Unambitious and non-competitive, they will put off getting to grips with anything that must be done; They are great procastinators.

The housewife loves her home and is hospitable. She likes to have her family round her and will be happy to sit for hours chatting over small incidents and domestic trivia.

They can, however, be fired up by somebody more forceful and get quite enthusiastic and do a job well – even push themselves to overwork.

Plain food is their thing, with plenty of starchy foods and dairy products; which of course is not a good thing given their tendency to be overweight.

They are lacking in confidence and back away from taking responsibility and fear failure. There is also a fear of the future and of misfortune.

One often sees a touch of Calc. Carb even in thin people, underlying whatever remedy is outstanding and an occasional dose will usually help in these cases.

Although this reads like a saga of negativity, they are actually lovely people to be with, as they will feed you cakes, trifles, and chat, but never be spiteful or willingly cause any trouble. They are not into spiteful gossip or character assassination – they are just nice easy people, happy to fit in and go along with the best.

If overworked they can throw everything up and opt out completely, and become completely unable to deal with anything financial. This kind becomes exhausted and feel they are losing their marbles and that everybody must have noticed it. Sleep becomes impossible as they lie in bed turning things over in their mind, not big problems but just silly little everyday things. When alone they will talk to themselves and to imaginary people about these little things. They go on and on about them and no amount of reassurance helps as they are unable to put their little worries into perspective.

In extremes they will have visions of murder, fire, rats, dogs and all manner of misfortunes, hysterical bouts of screaming and talk of the hereafter or they can just sit and refuse to speak.

Hepar Sulph

Hepar Sulph is a remedy that may be useful from time to time -particularly for patients who have had glandular problems and suppuration of one kind or another. They are prone to catarrh and offensive perspiration and ulceration.

They are very sensitive to cold and need to wear much clothing in cold weather; rooms must be overheated. Pain is another problem with them. They are oversensitive to pain which is always of the 'sticking' variety, and they are so sensitive to the slightest pain that they can even faint from it.

Mentally they are extremely irritable, angry, abusive and impulsive. They are afraid of their impulses, understandably so since the two constrasting impulses are to set fire to things and kill.

They are very quarrelsome, the least thing disturbs them; even somebody moving about the room infuriates them and they have a desire to jump up and kill them because they are so sensitive to the disturbance.

Nothing pleases them and they are continually dissatisfied – when they have got what they want, they are fed up with it, as they must have continual change.

Ignatia

Ignatia has been much maligned as being the remedy for hysterical women. What is termed hysterical behaviour is generally due to outbursts of irrational behaviour following an emotional upset or uncontrolable grief.

A true hysteric will manufacture situations in which she cn then have her 'fit of hysterics' and get the maximum manipulative mileage out of it. That is NOT Ignatia.

The Ignatia patient suffers from loss: loss of boyfriend, child, husband. She is very sensitive and will have headaches, sickness, weeping and trembling fits. Her grief has left her completely shattered. They tend sometimes to misplace their affection and then collapse with disappointment and grief if the affections are not returned. Occasionally a sensitive man will suffer in this way and there is no earthly reason why he should not have Ignatia. Men can and do become hysterical but their abandonment to grief is not so obvious. They want to be left to grieve alone and dwell on their troubles.

Like Argent.Nit., Ignatia has symptoms of trembling and agitation, but is more convulsive and the patient is sadder. Children may have convulsions after a fright or after being punished.

Hysterical paralysis may occur, but will usually pass off by itself. It is a contradictory remedy. Parts of the body which would be painful are better for pressure. If there is pain in the body, the patient is better for lying on the painful part.

Mild and sensitive and easily offended by nature, with

an inferiority complex, they feel unworthy and in the extreme believe themselves to be bad.

Sudden changes of mood occur and they change from laughter to crying and *vice versa* within seconds. Often they will complain of a lump in the throat, with yawning and sighing; and there is an aversion to tobacco smoke.

Contradiction can tip them from being weepy and sensitive to becoming completely unmanageable with prolonged hysterical paralysis and catalepsy with bending backwards and strange illusions.

Patients suffering from grief of many years standing can be helped enormously with this remedy.

Kali Brom.

Kali Brom is a remedy often useful in hyperactive children and teenagers. The whole picture in this remedy is restlessness and nervousness. They cannot keep still and must be constantly occupied. There is much twitching or clonic spasms and at school if anything is to be done they will start to tremble.

At night they worry, sometimes all night long, or nights may be interrupted with nightmares, screaming or grinding of teeth. In extreme cases there can be strabismus with fright or emotion.

In the adult there is a fear of people and fear of being alone. Uncontrolable weeping is common and constant complaining without proper reason. Alternatively, these patients can be mentally so exhausted that they will have loss of memory with a feeling as though there were a tight band round the head. In extreme cases there is suspicion, and delusions of persecution are common with muscular weakness, lack of coordination, ataxia and even paralysis. One strange phenomenon: they feel as though there is no ground beneath their feet; also numbness, with a peculiar symptom – as if there are needles pricking in the numbness.

Hallucinations of sight, sound and touch in the most extreme cases send these poor souls plunging down into melancholy and idiocy.

Kali Carb.

This remedy can be easily confused from a mental point of view with Hepar Sulph. The patient quarrels with everybody around him and is dissatisfied with his world but he is terrified of being alone, cannot bear to be alone in the house, can't get to sleep in case something dreadful happens – he is afraid it might burn down. He is also afraid of the future, ghosts and death.

Unable to bear draughts he must have all the windows closed. Cold will make him a martyr to neuralgias and his pains are sticking and burning, pain everywhere or just here and then there. He must wear lots of clothes and sweats easily in a cold sweat. One unusual thing about them is that they are very ticklish if you just touch them, especially the feet.

Mentally they are very very irritable and will quarrel with everybody over the least thing. I'm sure they would quarrel with themselves in an empty room, they are so irritable. Also they are dissatisfied with everything, house, job, friends, the lot.

Kali Phos.

Kali Phos is the front runner and remedy par excellance for a good old-fashioned nervous breakdown brought on by long periods of suffering, supressed anger, grief, and mental and physical overwork. It can be given to anybody with this condition until the indicated remedy has been selected.

This patient is physically and mentally worn out, discouraged, discontented, and sad, but can fly into tempers which leave them almost speechless. They are usually timid people, who when not ill, are easily upset when they hear bad news. They are anxious about the future, especially about their health, as they fear disease of any kind; even the smallest symptom sends them into a frenzy of worry, and they will brood on their condition. Reassurance does no good at all.

Anxiety is very prominent in bed at night and also when they are away from home. They can become very homesick. Fear is also prominent with fear of people, death, crowds, and even solitude.

These patients are very hurried in speech and action and extremely impatient and impetuous. They can become so worked up as to display contrary and hysterical behaviour. Often a woman will turn against her husband and family and even herself by refusing to eat.

Worn out by the fears and anxieties they will become indifferent, indolent and melancholic, with imaginings of dead people and all manner of frightful things.

Physically, these patients feel the cold and have an aversion to the open-air. One sided choreas, twitchings, jerkings and pulsations are common, as the whole organism is so disturbed.

47

Lac. Can.

Generally this patient is more often a woman than a man. She is forgetful, forgets what she was thinking, goes to fetch something from another room, and forgets what she went for, and has poor concentration.

Although she hates being alone, she has no fear of the dark which is odd, considering the imaginings that she has, and the anxiety she constantly suffers.

She is irresolute – always starting something and never finishing it, but since she feels hopeless and sees no point in living, she probably feels there is no point in finishing anything either. Nothing really seems worthwhile. Any minor ailment she believes to be a serious illness and in fact feels that she is just one mass of disease.

There are some distinctive physical feelings that arise from her anxiety and serve to feed it further. She feels she will stop breathing and that her heart has stopped beating. Floating feelings are common and very unnerving as she feels as though her feet are not on the ground; when in bed she feels as though she is floating above the mattress. Fears of snakes, falling, disease, and death are common.

The fear of snakes is so great that she has delusions and hallucinations and sees horrible sights. She feels as though she is infested with snakes and sees spiders and ugly faces. Strangely, the hallucinations only occur in the daytime, which is probably another reason why she is not afraid of the dark.

She cannot bear to be touched, and can't do with clothes touching her body. Even her fingers touching one another can be unbearable, and she will sit with her fingers splayed out.

Sensitivity to light and noise are common, as are cursing and swearing.

In spite of the forgetfulness, irresolution, and bizarre mental symptoms she manages to carry on from day to day doing her usual work. This, of course, is very difficult for the relatives to understand, as they feel she must be just saying these things for effect. Consequently, the poor soul will get no sympathy and probably no help either.

Lachesis

When well, the Lachesis type is intelligent, articulate and kind, with an incisive mind and loads of vitality. They are very loyal to their family and friends and expect the same loyalty in return. They are the kind of person who will stand up to be counted.

Aggravations usually occur in the spring, or on awakening in the morning and are generally left-sided. They can be prone to bursting headaches, palpitations and surges of heat in the body. The complexion may have a bluish tinge especially when they are flushed.

They hate tight clothing round the neck and will only wear open-necked clothes. They are also very fast eaters: the kind of person who chatters all through a meal and then finishes before everybody else. There is a tendency to jump from one subject to another and they will often tell you two or three tales at once, very often leaving sentences unfinished.

When unwell they will have an anxious expression with a 'bug eyed' look, even to the point of looking drunk, with stumbling speech or stammering.

There are signs of jealousy – particularly revengeful jealousy – and suspicion. As they progress downwards, they can become envious, conceited, revengeful and even maudlin. Well aware of others' weaknesses they use this to advantage to manipulate them. They seem to know how people are going to react to them and use this to advantage. In short, they become thoroughly unpleasant.

In extreme cases, they can believe they are being poisoned and refuse to eat. Their suspicious nature leads them to imagine that somebody is trying to get them committed. They feel that they are being compelled by the spirits to commit crimes and will confess to non-existent crimes or to other crimes that they have not committed.

Religious insanity is common, particularly in women. They feel that they have committed dreadful sins and will go on about them ad infinitum. Generally they have definite ideas about religion and can be either very pro or very anti and even bigoted in their beliefs.

In the maniacal stages, there is clairvoyance, clairaudiance, prophesying, violence, delerium and muttering. Eventually, when spent, the patient will contemplate suicide, but will become apathetic and just do nothing, having lost interest in everything.

Lycopodium

When well, the Lycopodium patient has quite a good opinion of himself and is sure in his own mind that he knows what is best. He manages to convey this attitude in a modest and reasonable fashion, so earning the respect of those around him. He is good at sorting out problems for other people as he likes to remain friendly with everyone and is able to remain detached. They are good people to have in the chair or performing some civic duty.

Because he knows what is right, he is not upset if somebody disagrees with him, he can just shrug it off as one of those things, they are obviously misguided.

He can be a difficult husband in that his wife may be climbing the walls trying to get him to understand her difficulties. He, after all, knows what is right and therefore the problem must be her's. He, however, is quite unaware that his attitude only makes the difficulties worse.

They usually look healthy, and wear very well but are inclined to neglect their health and can become prone to digestive and liver troubles, headaches, and renal calculi. They dislike becoming over-heated yet are sensitive to the cold and their symptoms usually start on the right side of the body, being worse in the late afternoon and early evening.

The first sign that something may be wrong is when they start to lose confidence. They will water up when meeting old friends or receiving a gift and can burst into tears when something makes them happy.

They become averse to meeting people, to their job

which they previously enjoyed, taking on new projects and being alone. Yet at the same time they need company not far away. There is no desire for conversation and a general air of 'can't be bothered, all I want is peace and quiet'. Friends, family and children all become an irritation to them.

They are afraid of making mistakes and forgetting things and with developing loss of confidence, cannot bring themselves to do anything, yet when pushed carry things off very well.

They wake feeling gloomy and sad and ponder on what can go wrong and imagine all kinds of gloomy scenarios. They may even beginto brood on religious subjects. Every thought has a dark side to it and negative feelings may become so deep that suicide seems the only answer.

Mercurius Sol.

The Mercury patient is hurried, restless, anxious and talks quickly, but for all this is mentally sluggish. They are forgetful and have difficulty when answering questions because they have forgotten the words they need.

When having something explained or receiving direction, they appear vacant as though what they are hearing is not registering – but will grasp it in the end.

Trembling and sweating are common, the sweating being worse at night in the warmth of the bed. It is difficult to get them to describe their feelings as they are determined to keep everything under control. They are impulsive and given to burst out into sudden fits of violent anger when that control slips, and they are very much aware that they have lost control, and fear they might hurt somebody or even themselves. They are easily startled and may react with an angry outburst out of proportion to the fright they have had.

Contradiction infuriates them to such a degree that they feel like killing the person who has contradicted them

If they progress into a demented state they become very suspicious and will pick quarrels with everybody and will even talk to themselves and grumble on at themselves and everybody around them.

Illusions are common, and they feel as though they are being tormented, and going insane. Certainly they can behave as though they are, and they will do stupid things, talk utter rubbish and generally act the goat.

On the other hand, they can become completely indifferent and appear not to care about anything.

In the maniacal stage, which is only likely to be seen in hospital since they will have been admitted long before this, they will be so afraid and try to run away, and not be able to recognise their own family.

Constantly talking and grumbling, they will spit, eat dirt, jump up and and down, throw off their clothes, become uncooperative and resistant to being touched. With all this they will not deliberately harm anybody, however alarming their behaviour seems.

These patients are worse in cold damp weather and extremes of temperatures and are always worse at night.

Roaring in the ears is a common symptom as are constricted feelings in the head. Mouth ulcers, halitosis, receding gums and offensive perspiration are all good physical pointers towards this remedy.

Nat. Ars.

The Nat. Ars. patient has a pale face with a yellowish cast and is usually thin. Either they have a large appetite with a good deal of stomach troubles or they may loathe food and feel sick after eating. They are very sensitive to the cold, as they feel cold and catch cold very easily.

Apprehensive, and anxious, they are always in a hurry and picky about every detail. If you contradict them they become absolutely furious.

They are particularly anxious later in the day and especially after midnight. They are afraid to go to bed, which isn't surprising since they have unpleasant anxious dreams and wake early, completely unrefreshed.

Fear is prominent in this remedy. There is a fear of people, particularly crowds, fear that something will happen, and fear of evil.

These patients have very active minds, consequently they are irritable and impatient, and can become hysterical. They will laugh and cry and talk nineteen to the dozen.

As the illness progresses, however, they become discontented, discouraged, and despairing. The mind becomes easily distracted, they become forgetful and dull. So exhausted do they become that they cannot think or work and just can't be bothered to do anything except lie down, which doesn't make them feel any better. So from being apparently hyperactive they end up by being dull and suspicious. They lose their social skills and have no desire to talk, and other peoples' conversations get on their nerves and make them irritable.

Their mental exhaustion can become so great that they have no joy in anything and appear to be complete imbeciles even though you may not see them in this condition as they will probably have been taking tranquillisers for some time.

Nat. Carb.

The Nat. Carb. patient in appearance has a pale face, often with yellowish patches of the forehead and face with a bluish tinge of the flesh around the eyes. There is a tendency to puffiness round the eyes and face. Some say they are stooping but I feel that it is more of a hang-dog demeanour.

They appear anxious, but although it is a fine point it is more nervousness than anything else. There is nervous excitement with internal and external trembling, and palpitations which make them exhausted. They suffer from nervous and physical exhaustion.

Forgetfulness is very marked as they cannot remember what they have read even a few minutes earlier, they can't add up, and forget what they were saying in mid-sentence. In extremes, there will be mental confusion.

Very anti-social, they don't want to mix with people, even their own immediate family. They have a definite aversion to people – and some people in particular they will take against as they find them distressing to be with. They feel cut off from their family, as though they are strangers to them.

Music makes them feel nervous, and they will cry when listening to it, and can even be driven to committing suicide by it. This is extreme of course and not often met with, but certainly, you won't find them listening to music. It is not surprising since they are very sensitive to noise. The slightest sound sounds very loud. Somebody opening a box of chocolates behind them in the cinema will make them very agitated. Although they may appear angered by small sounds of this nature it is definitely agitation. Very often they can be so annoyed that they will turn on the person making the noise with a sharp rebuke.

Sensitivity to bright lights can be very distressing for them as it makes the eyes actually painful, also the sense of taste may be over-developed and this too can be painful, or they may lose it altogether.

The reaction to temperature is important too – they are sensitive to the cold, can't stand draughts, so they usually wrap up well, but neither can they stand heat. In the summer they must sit in the shade, not just because of the heat but remember the light bothers them too.

Nat. Mur.

Nat. Mur. is the chronic of Ignatia. When Ignatia has helped and then ceases to work, Nat. Mur. will probably continue the improvement.

The similarities are laughing and crying alternatively, but whereas Ignatia changes from one to the other quickly, Nat Mur is more laughing when things are serious, and crying when they are funny. A fine distinction but worth looking for. They are also similar in their desire to be alone. Ignatia wants to be alone to be sad. Nat Mur is irritated by consolation or interference.

Nat. Mur. dwells on things, harbours grievances, doesn't want to forget old slights and insults, will cry in private and dislikes fuss.

Like Ignatia, this condition can be brought on by grief and unrequited love, but the subject is sadder and quieter than Ignatia.

Nat. Mur can become very depressed and frightened and thoroughly downhearted. This can alternate on another day by being happy and laughing.

There is an element of claustrophobia in this remedy too. Also a fear that somebody may be hiding in the house and she will search the house before going to bed (see Arsen Alb). She may dream of burglars etc.

They are unpredictable, independent and impulsive with bouts of unpredictable behaviour. The pattern is – irritable, unbearable – cross – then goes off for a good cry and is furious if offered consolation. She seems to be seeking consolation but furious when this is given.

The subject tends to be absent-minded and lacks concentration, as though they can't be bothered to think.

Noise, particularly scratching noises irritate them and they will suddenly flare up. Music may please them or it may irritate.

Usually these patients are fond of salt, but occasionally you will find one who never uses it. Generally, they are rather on the thin side, with a sickly or greasy complexion and given to spots on the forehead and hair line. However, some patients are not so thin and tend to retain fluid in the tissues, particulary when menstruating, and at this time will be at their worst, as the brain is further irritated by the waterlogging of the tissues.

Teenagers are liable to imagine they are in love with some unsuitable man and will mope around thoroughly miserable. Unfortunately, the same thing can happen to married women, particularly if they are disappointed in their marriage. The marriage is not what they expected, nor is the man they married and they will grieve for what they think they have lost. Imagine the distress of a Nat Mur patient married to an Aurum man. Small wonder that she falls in love with the man who comes to fit a new washing machine.

Nat. Phos.

The Nat. Phos. patient is similar in appearance to the Nat. Mur patient though generally thinner. Usually tall and spare and underweight for their size, they flush easily, the flushing usually confined to the cheeks.

Anxiety is a prominent feature here and they are worse in the evening, in bed, and before midnight, and on wakening in the morning. They worry about their health and future, and about little things, which they can become angry about.

Thoughts may be confused, particularly when it is necessary to concentrate, as they easily become distracted. Sometimes they are full of ideas and at others unable to gather their thoughts at all.

Everything they do is hurried and everybody else has to hurry with them and they will become quite hysterical with hurry.

They are inclined to vertigo whilst sitting and walking with a tendency to fall. Easily startled, they will jump at the slightest sound, and seem to be oversensitive to everything, especially pain.

There is a good deal of tension in these patients, the tension being so great that they will tremble and actually feel as though they are receiving shocks within the body.

Having become worn out with the hurry and tension, they will progress to a state of indifference: indifference to their family and their work. The brain becomes exhausted and they become suspicious, withdrawn and sad, even music makes them sad.

They are fitful sleepers, particularly between midnight

and 3 am and again around 5 a m. They are plagued with thoughts, anxious ones of course, and given to every kind of dream both anxious and sexual. So exhausted do they become, what with the hurry and worry of the day and broken nights, that they can be given to delusions, they imagine they are going to be ill, that they can see dead people, or that there is somebody creeping about in the house, and will actually hear their footsteps.

There is in the female an increased desire for sex, although one would expect them to be too worn out to bother, while in the male, there can be erections with no desire, or conversely,desire but no erections.

Their sensitivity to temperature is peculiar. They feel better in the warmth, but cannot stand to have sunshine on the head and have a tendency to be chilly. They hate draughts.

Nat. Sulph.

These patients are generally depressed and despairing, although there is an underlying anxiety. They are anxious about the future, and physically and mentally restless, and this is particularly marked in heavy weather or when thunder is in the air. Anxiety with irritability is common in the morning and evening but they are better in the middle of the day.

Sociability is certainly not their strong point, as they dislike talking to people and being talked to and hate crowds, of which they are afraid. They are oversensitive, easily frightened, and suspicious, particularly when being questioned and can become violently angry. Even music will not cheer them up; on the contrary, it makes them sad.

There is a definite loathing of life with indifference, forgetfulness and laziness being very marked, but with all this gloominess they can become hysterical. In the later stages, they will become determined to commit suicide and in these cases talking will do little good as they are suspicious of what you say to them and will probably have to be physically restrained from actually harming themselves.

Photophobia, noises in the ears, palpitations with trembling and hypersensitivity to pain are good physical pointers when choosing between the other Natrum salts. Although stuffy rooms aggravate them they can also be chilly, particularly in the evening, when they will want something warm to put on.

Nux Vomica

When well the Nux Vomica type is sympathetic and patient with the emotions well in check.

They are generally quietly spoken, clear minded and diplomatic. However they tend to be workaholics, competitive, ambitious and successful at what they do. They are the busy, hard-working people who will always fit in one more job. They appreciate good workmanship themselves and in others and expect everybody to do as well as they.

Because they are super competent they feel that the way they do things must be right; their will hover over their employees and family, instructing them how to do their jobs, and become thoroughly exasperated with anyone who prefers to do things by their own methods, even though the results are just as good.

This of course puts enormous strain on them and they develop an irritable character. As they have too many jobs on the go, small details will irritate them and they develop the 'don't bother me with that now' syndrome and begin to feel their associates are incompetent. People around them tend to stop taking any responsibility because they know any decision they make will be wrong anyway; and so the strain builds up.

They enjoy good food and have a tendency to overindulge not only in food, which must be well presented, but wines, spirits, cigarettes, coffee and in certain cases drugs, all of which help to calm them.

Physically, they are prone to digestive upsets . They are chilly yet sweat easily, disturbed by the slightest noise and tend to have broken nights and never get into a really good zizz.

They are sensitive to noise, draughts and smells which can send them into irritable outbursts. They cannot stand being contradicted – even the slightest contradiction will make them furious – and they can be generally very difficult to live with.

Their physical ailments tend to be spasmodic. The digestive troubles are common and they are prone to twitching, neuralgias, trembling and, in the extreme, paralysis and convulsions.

If his secretary tidies his desk, or his wife moves his books and papers about at home, he becomes very irritable and if something is in his way he will just plough on, kicking it aside regardless of the fact that it may be broken or spoiled.

His sensitivity to pain is so great that he can be driven to suicide by it.

Phosphorous

The Phosphorous patients when well are bright, attractive, articulate, glowing personalities who have to give and receive affection. Usually they have plenty of ideas but have not the stamina to carry them through. They are sympathetic and comforting to friends in need but again cannot sustain their interest for too long.

Unfortunately, if overtaxed and overworked they can become very ill indeed and become mentally and physically exhausted.

Sleep is essential and they are always better after a good sleep when they can get it. They become very excitable, which keeps them awake at night. Light, smells, noise and the least touch can excite them, and sleep becomes literally a nightmare, with visions of horrible old faces in the room with them.

They become anxious when alone, with a great fear of the night and of death. They are always afraid something will happen and have feelings of fear in the stomach; and fear in thundery weather.

Physically there is trembling, paralytic weakness, with inability to walk properly. Prolonged muscle spasms and jerking in the muscles are common, as is Formication.

In more extreme cases they become weeping, sad hypochondriacs and lose interest in friends, family, their surroundings and even their children.

There is a state of dazed stupefaction with the inability to think or answer questions. Any mental effort gives them a headache. Dejection and gloom are the order of the day.

Near manic episodes may occur with fury, violence, wild talking and delirium, and drunken staggering. When in this state noise, even music, will drive them wild.

The Phosphorous patient feels the cold and is always better for rest and warmth. They suffer dreadful headaches and eye problems, which are always better for heat.

Platina

The Platina patient is invariably female, her troubles brought on by shock, disappointment and long periods of stress. She is anxious, moody, sulky and crying. Trembling is a prominent physical feature, coupled with paralytic weakness, compressive feelings in the head and numbness in the scalp.

She attaches too much weight to trivial matters and makes mountains out of molehills, working herself up into hysteria. She is restless and excitable, never still. These hysterical bouts can reach the manic stage or she may relapse into melancholy.

This poor lady is arrogant, haughty, with overwhelming pride, over-estimates herself and is quite sure that others are inferior to her. She feels taller physically than others, people and objects appearing small to her. She may go so far as to claim important antecedents or embellish her relatives with important positions. She is contemptuous of everybody and everything.

There is a great fear of losing her husband, that he will go out and never come back. The most well-trained and well-behaved husband, who has never put a foot wrong, can be driven away by her lack of confidence. It is not so much jealousy as the fear he may be lost to her.

Very amorous, she will talk about sex and can be quite vulgar, however unsuitable the occasion; sexual perversions are quite common.

She can be quite noisy to live with as there is a tendency to whistle, sing and dance, laughing at sad things and at serious situations. She is not awfully keen on her children

69

either and can be disparaging, as she sees them as small and insignificant, not at all in keeping with her grand status.

Platina is worth considering in cases of paranoia and religious mania though. Not inclined to suicide for all that she is disenchanted with the world, she is terrified of dying, which she is expecting to do at any time.

Pulsatilla

The Pulsatilla patient, generally a female, usually looks quite well, even when she is ill, and is rounded, soft and inclined to plumpness. Again this remedy can be needed in the male.

She is nervous, fidgity and changeable, yet tractable, and easily led. Irritability is there but not irascibility.

Public opinion is very important to her as she is touchy and easily feels slighted and can be full of self pity. Relief is gained by crying, which comes easily. She will cry when she is telling the therapist about her feelings, and go off feeling much better. The sun won't be out for long however since she craves attention and praise constantly, and life being what it is she is not going to get it. Consequently, she will soon be feeling sorry for herself again.

Although fidgity and irritable, she can sit silently and need coaxing to talk sometimes.

This patient likes sex very much and with patience, and given the right circumstances, will say so even though she seems shy. In fact, her sexual desire can be so strong as to be classed as nymphomania.

There is a fear of the dark, and fear of being alone and the fear is felt in the stomach.

Some physical symptoms are important to take into consideration here: vertigo, one sided congestive headaches, or migraine, feeling suffocated in a warm room, and retention of fluid in the tissues. All these symptoms are worse at the time of the periods, with hot flushes and a fear of going mad.

Obsessiveness is strong in this patient. She can be

determined that certain foods are bad for her and the human race in general. Being easily led as well as obsessive, she is a ripe candidate for cults of one kind or another.

Religious obsessions are common too, not mania exactly, but more likely an unusual religious group, or a misinterpretation of the scriptures, which she is determined to live by.

Strangely, this rather soft sensitive patient can at times be extremely impolite and use some very bad language. Jealousy is also there but is not as obvious as in some other remedies such as Lachesis.

In extremes, this patient will become suicidal, drowning being the method of choice.

Dr.Borland, in his *Childrens Types*, mentions a Pulsatilla type which is slimmer. This type of Pulsatilla is harder to spot in an adult and will be found amongst the women who appear much younger than their years with the expressions and behaviour of a young teenage girl. Very often this type will look for an older man to marry, as she probably has not had a satisfactory relationship with her father.

Sepia

Sepia is again another predominantly female remedy, although occasionally men will need it. In many ways it is similar to Nat. Mur, and it complements it, so they may be given together if necessary or, even better, Sepia to follow Nat Mur when Nat Mur has failed.

The Sepia patient gives the impression of being dull, heavy, and sallow, often with a smooth round, doughy face. Brown patches may also appear on the skin of the face.

The expression is dull and she appears to be intellectually dull. This can be misleading as she can be as quick as anybody when well. She is, however, dull company, with little sense of humour, which isn't surprising since she feels that there is nothing for her in living.

Everything seems strange and unreal, even her family and friends. There is a feeling that she doesn't love her family. She knows she loves them but doesn't feel as though she does. There is a paucity of emotion – a cut-off feeling, and she has no interest in her husband, so there are usually sexual and marital problems to contend with. All but the most saintly husbands will have probably started to look elsewhere by the time she presents for treatment.

This poor lady sits about, avoids work, is sad and quiet and disinclined to talk. She will hardly answer her family when they try to talk to her and cannot be stirred to any enthusiasm for anything. The only excitement she shows is when she is suicidal.

She dreads being alone in spite of the fact that company

annoys her, as do light , noise and cooking smells.

Hysterical bouts are common and she will alternate between being weepy and tractable, to being obstinate, vindictive, and unpredictable. Her family cannot rely on her to do anything as not only does she not want to, she will make mistakes in anything she does.

There can be eccentric behaviour and she will be sarcastic, spiteful, and rude to her friends and relations in particular, but anybody will do, although she herself is easily offended and quick to moan on about her troubles.

Menstruation seems to magnify her symptoms and she will feel as though she is going mad. Fancies can occur of ghosts of which she is afraid and she is given to feeling that the spirits of her relatives are about although she does not see them; and she is quite likely to join a spiritualist group or something of that kind.

Her contemporaries must agree with her, as she gets very annoyed with anybody who takes the opposite point of view. She will brook no argument.

Silica

The Silica personality is pleasant, good tempered and straight-forward, apparently tractable, though underneath they can be stubborn and quietly wilful.

They are not pushy and will shun the limelight yet would like recognition. They will allow themselves to be over-shadowed and have difficulty in making friends. There is a dislike of arguments which they try hard to avoid and if involved in any unpleasantness they will only think of what they should have said when it is too late.

Criticism destroys them as they feel unable to stick up for themselves, and contradiction upsets them too though they may not show it. This makes them angry with themselves, but only occasionally will they show it. They are very insecure and do not expect to succeed, putting themselves down at every opportunity and there is a definite fear of failure or that they have never done anything worthwhile.

They are, however, clear minded, honest, reliable, often gifted with E.S.P. When feeling reasonably secure, such as in their own home, they can be bright and cheerful, but tend to be restless and embark on unnecessary jobs. They can have set ideas and once having embarked on a course will stick at it and do it well and even overdo it being very concientious and tidy by nature.

They seem emotionally young for their age as though they have never learned to protect themselves emotionally and there is a terrible fear of appearing in public, especially if it be necessary to speak. They will tremble so much it is almost impossible to get the words out.

When ill, they dislike being touched, spoken to or looked at. All they want is peace and quiet. They do not want to go out as meeting people is so disturbing that it isn't worth the trouble. They become irritable, sad, despondent, and bad-tempered if aroused. There is fear of burglars who they are sure are trying to break in and religious melancholy.

Physically, they are prone to hard swellings of the glands, calcareous nodules, cracked skin, particularly around the nails and finger ends, hard boils and carbuncles. Silica is well recommended for use in all these conditions. There is a tendency to sweat about the head and offensive foot sweat, and being of a chilly disposition they prefer warm, dry conditions and physical comfort.

Much is made of the 'weary willy' appearance of these patients, but I have to say that there are plenty of patients in need of Silica who look very well indeed and who are in physically good health.

Staphisagria

The patient needing this remedy is the type of person who is excitable, easily angered but suffers in silence. Their whole life is spent in suppressing the feelings of anger and hurt; They never discuss their feelings or problems. They are easily angered by real and imaginary insults and should they suffer any unfair treatment will bottle it all up, allowing the anger to seethe away beneath the surface. They feel they must control their emotions or disintegrate completely.

This unhealthy attitude will naturally have dire consequences which can result in poor memory, even loss of memory, sleeplessness, trembling, mistakes at work, and complete mental and physical exhaustion. They can be so beside themselves with supressed rage that they are unable to speak and eventually become depressed, with no will to make any effort, just wanting to be alone.

The head feels compressed and there is a feeling as if there were a ball in the forehead and an empty feeling at the back of the head. Hypersensitivity to noise, light and smells is common.

A lot of time is given to thinking about sex, which can so excite the female sexual organs that a state of nymphomania is possible, while the male who masturbates a good deal will be impotent, despite his ardent desire.

This is a good remedy to consider when dealing with such cases as people who have been put down within the family or at work and actually insulted. They have festered away for years until eventually presenting for treatment depressed, aphonic, and shaking.

The suppression of their emotional energy disturbs them physically, causing pain in the bones, bowels and joints.

Sulphur

Sulphur is an amazing remedy: with it almost every symptom is possible, so wide a range does it cover. In chronic illness, it can be very useful when the picture is muddled. A dose of Sulphur will alter the case and it will then be possible to select the fitting remedy. Most people have a streak of Sulphur in their make-up so it can be used from time to time during any course of treatment to move the case along, especially when the indicated remedy ceases to act.

There are two basic Sulphur types: the vigorous and the more indolent type. The most well known type of Sulphur is the one with a poor physique with thin legs, narrow chest, lacking in vitality, low and miserable. Generally scruffy, they adopt a life style which affords the least possible effort. They will spend their lives theorising about anything, very often politics and the merits of various religions, etc., etc. and will spend hours putting the world to rights in theory but not in practice. They feel weak and tired all the time and hate standing up – they find it impossible to stand for long and will lean on anything handy.

Tatty clothes are the norm and washing is well down their list of priorities. They will buy second hand clothes which they will don in bizarre combinations and think that they look just fine. So we see here the Hippie Culture as a prime example. Material things are shunned and they will often opt out of society and be quite happy drawing social security.

On the other hand, there is the stronger Sulphur type –

better built and with plenty of go. Generally selfish and inconsiderate, they are materialistic and want their own way. They are big collectors and hate parting with anything or sharing with others and they can be very tactless. This type has a big ego and will put big schemes into operation which others are expected to carry out – but will take all the glory. This Sulphur type is usually male. He likes to make money and on the one hand is tight-fisted, but on the other he can't resist flashing it. The scrapman with a yacht is the way I think of him. Everything he owns he thinks is the best so he will be boastful. They can also be impatient and argumentative. You will notice this in teenagers who want something and they must have it at once.

Less obvious is the intellectual, who is to some extent a mixture of these two basic types: the rather untidy professor who collects vast quantities of information and produces prodigious works, who can blind any seminar with facts and statistics. His house will be full of books, papers, sea shells, works of art, while the more ordinary man will collect road signs, railway signals, pieces of cars and motor bikes and is quite likely to have a bicycle on the kitchen table which he started to rebuild last year.

Female Sulphurs are less obvious, a sort of paler edition if you like. She will hoard bits of curtain material, wool, cooking pots that she never uses anymore, bottoms and lids that don't fit each other and so on. Nothing is thrown away.

Because they are full of ideas and spend so much time on them they can be very inventive and come up with some very good ideas – flashes of inspiration is probably the best description. Sometimes they are ideas that turn out to be very useful indeed. This leads many of them to believe that education is unnecessary for them as they have plenty of ideas anyway.

When mentally ill they will lose their concentration

and become forgetful and worried. All their traits become accentuated, especially silly ideas about religion. They will meditate and pray for hours on end and believe that they have done many wrong things for which they will never be forgiven and wish they could die.

There are many outstanding physical symptoms, a few of which I will mention: skin problems of every conceivable kind which are worse for warmth and worse from washing, with temporary relief from scratching; early morning diarrhoea which smells foul; hunger for tasty foods and sweets (especially hungry at 11 a.m. – and they are always thirsty); catarrhal problems which are common and can be foul smelling, and flushes of heat which are common too. The physical symptoms of Sulphur are so vast however that it is much easier to select the remedy from the mental and general charactaristics. The really outstanding things about them are the acquisitiveness and the untidiness, this combination must always lead one to think of Sulphur.

Thuja

The Thuja patient looks thoroughly unwell. He is pale with a waxy complexion, often with a yellowish tinge.

This remedy works wonders if you can spot it out, but it is difficult. The patient is perfectly fine with strangers, pleasant and co-operative but not so nice at home, so it will be helpful to consult a relative about their normal behaviour within the family.

They are violently irritable, jealous and will pick quarrels all the time, and are positively 'hateful' and they feel like that too. It seems that they want to be cruel to their loved ones. There is a tendency to get a bee in the bonnet, which no amount of reassurance will shift.

They will ponder for ages over small jobs and minor problems, probably because they can't think clearly, as they make mistakes when reading and writing. Sometimes they speak slowly as though they are waiting for every word to come to mind and will often not be able to say what they want because they can't find the right word.

In the extreme they will feel as though they are being followed, or someone is beside them, or they are being influenced by a superior power, and even that their sense has separated from their body.

When these patients are undergoing drug therapy and not experiencing the extreme symptoms, it is important closely to question the relatives about their personality prior to this stage, as very often the patient will not tell you himself. Helpful here are some physical symptoms: usually there are warts and moles on the body, possibly combined with skin problems, headaches, rheumatic troubles, perspiration which smells of onions, a wooden feeling in the legs,and a sensation as if there is secretion moving about in the abdominal cavity, or that they might break into pieces.

METALS

Nowadays we are subjected to more metallic poisoning than we were in the past. Although lead has been banned in paints, we still breathe it and eat it in our food. I hope that this environmental problem is now well in hand and the quantities we ingest will gradually be reduced over the next decade. Copper was thought to be safer for water pipes, but even so in soft water areas the hot water can absorb copper which can cause imbalances in the body.

People have become alert to the possibility of aluminium poisoning, but many catering establishments still use aluminium for some processes: Many indigestion remedies contain aluminium.

Although many of the metals cause recognised physical problems they can also cause mental problems, and very often the patient will be dubbed neurotic.

Mercury fillings upset some people both mentally and physically and where this is causing a problem they should be removed and replaced with light cured composite or porcelain crowns.

All metallic poisoning deranges the body metabolism, causing the processing of minerals and vitamins to be altered. The Amino Acids chain can also be interfered with. However, we are straying into the realms of the dietician here and anybody who is suffering from these conditions, would, along with the homoeopathic treatment, benefit enormously from consulting a well qualified Dietary Therapist who understands exactly the supplementation necessary to help them over the detoxification period and speed recovery.

Homoeopathic treatment of metallic poisoning is best begun by giving either a potency of the offending metal, or one of the antidotes. I usually give the 30c potency for 3–5 days once a fortnight, maybe moving to the higher potency 1M after six weeks.

Sometimes, one of the antidotes fits the symptoms better than the metal itself and, if this be the case, use one of them. This, it must be stressed, is only a first-aid treatment. The offending cause must be removed whenever possible for any dietary or supplementary treatment to work. This does not mean in the case of copper that all the plumbing must be removed, but care should be taken only to use water from the cold tap, as used to be the case with lead. Copper certainly doesn't cause the same problems as lead used to do.

ALUMINA

The person is sad, with no expectation of being cured. There is anxiety, with fear of having committed a crime; bored, apprehensive with no desire to work, or even to talk – finds it exhausting. Time seems to pass too slowly for them. They seem to be hasty but take a long time to do a job. They can become depressed especially on wakening. There is a fear of knives or a fear of blood.

Forgetfulness is common with mistakes in writing and reading. Sometimes timid and sometimes forceful and they sometimes feel larger than they are.

These patients when really ill can feel suicidal yet are disgusted with the idea of it. They are afraid of what they might do.

These mental symptoms can be easily confused with a number of other remedies so some physical symptoms are of help here, especially those of the alimentary tract.

The appetite of these patients can be irregular, sometimes too hungry and then no desire to eat; alumina always be considered in cases of bulimia. There is also in some patients a strong aversion to animal foods, especially meat, but there is a strong desire for vegetables and fruits. Often they have a sweetish taste in the mouth. Potatoes often don't agree with them and will give them bitter risings. Anything they eat that doesn't agree with them will start them coughing and they will sometimes complain of a feeling like a splinter in the throat.

Colic is a common complaint too and can usually be relieved by a hot water bottle. The intestines are inactive and they are often plagued with constipation and may even have no desire to perform. The stool is hard, knotty and painful and covered with mucous. Aluminium is antidoted by Bryonia, Camphor, Chammomilla and Ipececuana.

CUPRUM (COPPER)

These patients are anxious and tearful, alternating with silly behaviour – acting the goat – and fits of convulsive laughter. They can also be compliant or sometimes obstinate. They are unfit for any work but afraid of being idle. There is restlessness wih a desire to escape, and fits of anguish.

In extreme cases they will become delirious and pretend to be doing a job of some kind, accompanied by singing, or on the other hand may become morose and lose all sense.

The appetite is not so capricious as in the other two metals, but they too have a sweetish, or metallic taste – or salty which the other two do not have. Everything tastes watery and there is a desire for cold food rather than hot. Drinking milk will provoke a flow of watery saliva.

Growing cramps in the stomach and constant risings in the oesophagus are common in all these remedies.

Abdominal pain with anxiety, all sensations are sensitive to touch, the colic making them cry out.

Constipation which makes them feel very hot or on the other hand diarrhoea with blood in it, helps to distinguish from the other two remedies.

Cuprum is antidoted by Belladonna, Chamomilla, China, Conium, Dulcamara, Cicuta, Hepar Sulph, Ipececuana, Merc. Sol, Nux Vomica.

As will be seem from reading through these remedies, there are many similarities between them. Also in common they have kidney symptoms of a non-specific kind where no proper diagnosis can be found. Cloudy, turgid urine with casts, and sometimes blood have been known to occur.

One such patient of mine presented with no specific kidney ailment. She had had every investigation known to man and had been told her kidneys were failing and nothing was to be done. In conversation however, she happened to mention that one bright medical student had asked her if she cooked or worked with aluminium. She had a mouthful of dental amalgam and one gold filling. These fillings were tested and found to have a high level of electrical activity.

The fillings were removed and she was given a potency of dental amalgam along with supplements of Selenium. She is now in good health and leading a normal life in spite of some irreversible kidney damage in her left kidney.

Herein lies the difficulty in spotting these metal poisonings, as very often only one part of the body may be affected, so it is necessary to read well in to the Materia Medica of these remedies sometimes to be able to treat sucessfully, as all homoeopathic similia to her condition had failed. Once the existing cause had been removed, treatment went on apace.

A similar scenario applies to the extremities of the

body. In all these metal poisonings it is possible to ob-
serve pullings drawings, pain, partial tendency to and in
some cases apparently permanent paralysis of many parts.
Co-ordination problems are common as is stumbling
gait, weakness of limbs and clonic spasms.

PLUMBUM (Lead)

These patients are timid, restless, anxious and liable to
exaggerate their condition. They have no taste for work
which leaves them mentally exhausted. They are dull,
stupid and miserable and very much averse to company.
They can become delerious and have a fear of being
assassinated.

All their symptoms are changeable and non-specific,
no doubt leading to them being taken for neurotic com-
plainers. They may have a right facial twitch and even
epilepsy. One unusual symptom to look for is a trembling
tongue. There can be wasting of the limbs and paralysis
from time to time of various parts of the body.

Tension in the abdomen with colic and radiating abdominal pain. Persistent constipation with hard stools
like sheep dung which are passed with cramping feelings
in the belly and they may even break out in a cold sweat
when passing a stool. Abdominal pain will sometimes
make them cry out and they feel as though they must
stretch. Liver problems and ileocaecal problems are common too in these patients.

Their appetite can be capricious with either anorexia or
excessive hunger with a great desire for fried foods and
bread. Sticky saliva with deranged taste which may be
sweetish, bitter or metallic with a foul acid taste in the
throat. Lead is antidoted by Alumina, Arsen.alb.,
Antim.Crud., Belladonna, Hepar.Sulph., Nux.Vom., Opium,
Petroleum, Platina, Zinc.

DRUG ADDICTION

Many patients who present for Psychotherapy these days have in the past taken drugs, or smoked cannabis. In these cases, I would give them a homoeopathic potency of the drug in question at the commencement of treatment and then wait a few weeks before taking the case.

When this option is not available the best course is to administer either Sulphur 1M or Nux Vomica 1M whichever fits the symptoms best. Some people use what is called the scrubbing technique, giving alternatively Sulphur 30 and Nux Vomica 30 one dose weekly for alternate weeks. Either method seems to work equally well, though perhaps dyed in the wood and dedicated addicts probably do better on the scrubbing method.

Cannabis and Opium are still available in Homoeopathic potency at the time of writing but are under review and may not in the future be available in the lower potencies.

However, we must not overlook the allergic component in these cases as mentioned elsewhere in this book, as more rapid progress will be made if the addictive foods are dealt with. With regard to potentising other drugs, some Homoeopathic Pharmacies are willing to do this and others are not, but certainly if these services are available it is easier to treat the patient when they have had a potency of the offending drug. The same principle applies to prescribed drugs, when a patient is undergoing psychotherapy as it helps them to withdraw with much less trauma.

A new label 'the addictive personality' has recently been suggested. I don't believe there is any such thing. Chemical imbalances can be brought on by malabsorption and malnutrition and there is no doubt that some people need far more of some particular nutrients to remain in balance than the statutory recommended daily dose. These can generally be spotted out by a Nutritionalist or Clinical Ecologist and many cases of aberrant behaviour have been rectified by these Therapists.

Once again, we come back to the allergic patient. Allergies can be brought on by physical and mental trauma and very often a complete cure is not possible without treating these patients for this problem. Many allergic patients cannot be properly treated without Psychotherapy and vice-versa. If they can have the correct homoeopathic remedy as well, so much the better, and as the patients mental symptoms change, so must the homoeopathic remedy change to match.

Luckily, homoeopathic treatment combines well and does not interfere with any of the other alternative therapies, so it behoves us to give the patient every available chance to get well. Some of the complicated cases respond well to homoeopathy and counselling alone, but addiction is generally much more difficult to deal with and combining therapies at various stages of the long-term treatment is even better.

CONCLUSION

In conclusion then it is never a good idea to look at mental illness in isolation but rather to investigate physical symptoms at the same time.

There are many conditions that can mimic or contribute to mental illness, such as Candida Albicans infestation, Hypoglycaemia, M.E., Thyroid imbalance, food and chemical allergy, dietary imbalance with nutritional deficiences and metallic poisoning.

Neither should we overlook chemical poisoning with materials such as pesticides and prescribed drugs. In the cases of drug addiction and alcoholism it should be borne in mind that these patients will more than likely in the past have been suffering from masked allergies which are addictive in nature. If possible these must be dealt with for permanent progress to be made. An example of this could be a patient who was a sugar addict and hypoglaecaemic with upswings in well-being having eaten the sweet stuffs followed very shortly by a downswing in well-being. Grain and yeast products can have a similar effect.

Small wonder then that some patients begin to display neurotic behaviour. They feel ill and know they are ill yet all tests prove negative. They are understandably prescribed tranquilisers and anti-depressants with no success. These people are such a worthwhile challenge and much detective work is needed along with the help of different therapies before complete success is achieved.

I had a patient recently who had dizzy spells and fell about while doing her housework and during the night would completely pass out. Neurological investigations were of no avail, nor were the administration of Homoeopathic treatment, or Chiropractic, or large doses of Valium, which she was still taking. One day she said to me 'Well, if you can do nothing for me, can you do something for my dog?' To cut a long story short, the dog slept in her room because it regularly vomited in the night. She would get up, clean up the mess and spray the room with air freshener. The following day a chemical carpet cleaner was applied and then hoovered up, whereupon she passed out. If it had not been for that casual conversation neither I nor the best brains in the neurological department could have helped her. She cured herself by throwing out all air fresheners, carpet cleaners and the like.

Another case of chemical sensitivity was a lady who on the face of it was becoming agoraphobic. If she got into her car to go shopping she felt unreal and had to turn back and the same thing applied to her job. Homoeopathy and Psychotherapy made no improvement nor did lead allergy testing and desensitisation help much either. I walked to her car with her and as she opened the door I smelled a strong smell of perfume. On the dashboard was a stick on air freshener. This was discussed as a possible source of the problem and she rang me a week later to say she had thrown it out along with toilet fresheners and was now very well thank you.

All the aforementioned conditions are things that we must take into consideration in the age in which we live; and all are subjects for books in themselves. So it behoves us to leave no stone unturned when dealing with mental illness.

This book has been written with Psychotherapists in mind. It will be helpful to practitioners of other therapies who often find their patients have some mental difficulties, particulary therapists who practice counselling. The use of the correct homoeopathic remedy will liberate the psyche of the patient and facilitate a quicker cure. Even physical therapists will benefit by its use as many patients supress mental pain which then becomes locked into the muscular and skeletal system. Rheumatism can be helped by using the correct homoeopathic remedy, as certain types of personality with particular mind sets are more prone to rheumatism than others.

It is not recommended that people who have no training attempt to treat serious mental disorders without the help of a qualified therapist; on the other hand, mild imbalances can successfully be treated within a family setting. Often a parent or spouse can be very perceptive in these matters and can help to balance the personality by the judicious use of the correct remedy.

Suggested Reading

Portraits of Homoeopathic Medicines: Psychological Analyses of Selected Constitutional Types Vols 1 & 2 and *Portrait of Indifference Supplement to Vol 2*; Catherine Coulter: North Atlantic Books

Not All in the Mind; Richard Mackarness – London: Pan Books

Homoeopathic Remedies for Children; Phillis Speight – Saffron Walden: Health Science Press

Studies of Homoeopathic Remedies; Douglas Gibson: Beaconsfield Publishers Ltd

The Homoeopathic Treatment of Illness; Dr Trevor Smith: Thorsons Publishers Ltd

Useful Addresses

British Homoeopathic Association, 27a Devonshire Street, London W1N 1RJ.

Hahnemann Society, Humane Education Centre, Bounds Green Road, London N22 4EU.

Homoeopathic Development Foundation, Harcourt House, 19a Cavendish Square, London W1M 9AD.

Society of Homoeopaths (Register of Homoeopaths), 2 Artisan Road, Northampton NN1 4HU. Institute for Neurophysiological Psychology (for OBD treatment), 4 Stanley Place, Chester, Cheshire.

Institute of Allergy Therapists (Register of Allergists), Llangwyryfon, Aberystwyth, Dyfed.

Donald M Harrison B.A. (Hons), B.Sc., M.R.Pharm.S. (Homoeopathic Chemist) Ffynnonwen Natural Therapy Centre, Llangwyryfon, Aberystwyth, SY23 4EY

National Institute of Medical Herbalists, 41 Hatherley Road, Winchester, Hants.

Ainsworth's (Homoeopathic Chemists), 38 New Cavendish Street, London W1M 7HL.

Nelsons (Homoeopathic Chemists), 7a3 Duke Street, London W1.

Sheila Harrison R.G.N., Ffynnonwen Natural Therapy Centre, Llangwyryfon, Aberystwyth, Dyfed.